Federal Pharmacy Law Review for the MPJE

by Sarah Fichuk, Pharm.D., BCPS

NAPLEX®, MPJE®, and NABP® are federally registered trademarks owned by the National Association of Boards of Pharmacy (NABP®). This book is in no way endorsed, sponsored, or authorized by NABP®.

Printed in the United States of America

First Printing, 2012

ISBN 978-0615667812

Straight A's Publishing

www.StraightAsPublishing.com

Table of Contents

Section One: Introduction

Test Overview

- Online registration at www.nabp.net
- Computer-based test
- Adaptive technology selects the next question based on the answers to your previous questions
- No distinction between federal and state law (answer according to the strictest rule)
- 2 hours for 90 questions
- 75 scored questions
- 15 pretest questions
- Scored questions are not identified
- Minimum passing score is 75 in a range of 0–100
- Scaled score (compares your score to the minimum acceptable score)
- Cannot change an answer once it has been confirmed
- Cannot go back and review questions
- All questions must be answered in order
- Cannot skip questions
- Scores are available online at www.nabp.net within 7 business days (usually in 2-3 business days)

Federal Laws and Rules Tested on the MPJE®

- Federal Food, Drug and Cosmetic Act
- Federal Controlled Substance Act
- Poison Prevention Packaging Act
- Pseudoephedrine Laws

How to Study

I recommend that you make sure you read the sections **Make Sure You Know These!** and **Test Objectives** prior to reading through this book and your state specific study materials. That way you know what information to pay special attention to while studying. Everything is important, but there are certain things you must know.

I suggest you read through the chapters at least **3** times, then go back to the **Make Sure You Know These!** list and make sure you can answer each one as if it were a question.

Particularly focus on all the information in the controlled substances section. Read that section again just prior to taking the test. It would be better to be over-prepared rather than underprepared. This is one of the most important tests of your career.

When to Schedule Your Exams

I recommend focusing on only one exam at time, either the NAPLEX® or the MPJE®. You will probably need a minimum of a week to study for the MPJE®, if not two weeks. So keep that in mind when scheduling your exams.

Actually Taking the Test

There will be answers like "1 and 2," "2 only," and "1, 2 and 3."

Read each question carefully. Do not read too much into the question or try to overanalyze—think in straightforward terms and go with your first choice when reading the answers.

Do not rush through each question. You have plenty of time to take the test—over a minute for each question—and some will be easy and straightforward, so don't panic about time. Some questions, you have to guess at, so don't get discouraged.

Warning/Disclaimer

This book is not intended to be comprehensive review of all pharmacy law. Many of the rules and laws applicable to the practice of pharmacy were **NOT** included because the author felt they were unlikely to be on the MPJE®. This book is a study guide to help pharmacists and pharmacy students pass the federal law questions on the MPJE®. It is intended to be a supplement to the law class taken in pharmacy school.

If the reader has concerns over a statement made in this book or has further questions, the reader should read the actual law referenced.

A word of caution: Even if you have worked retail as a technician for years, you still need to study to pass this test. The pharmacy you worked at may not have been following the law as written.

Test Objectives

Federal and State Controlled Substance Acts and Regulations

- Definitions of controlled substances
- Who registers with DEA and DPS and how
- Storage requirements for controlled substances
- What records must be maintained
- Central record keeping requirements and restrictions
- Obtaining, executing, and storing DEA order forms
- Returning controlled substances to supplier
- Disposing expired or contaminated controlled substances
- Prescription requirements for Schedule II–V
- Refill requirements for Schedule II–V
- Emergency refill requirements for Schedule III–V
- Partial dispensing of Schedule II and Schedule III–V
- Emergency oral order of Schedule II
- Federal "transfer warning" statement
- OTC sale of Schedule V products
- Schedule II prescription requirements and exceptions
- Criteria to place a drug in the five schedules
- Recognizing commonly used controlled substances and their schedules
- Reporting theft/loss to DEA and DPS
- Employee screening
- Procedures for closing a business
- Legal use of methadone
- Methadone to treat addiction
- Using Subutex® or Suboxone®
- Physicians' designated agents
- Faxed Schedule II prescriptions

Federal and State Food, Drug, and Cosmetic Acts

- Definitions
- Adultered
- Misbranded
- Registration requirements for manufacturers and distributors
- Illegal pharmacist acts under the Durham-Humphrey Amendments
- Requirements for manufacturers' labels
- How long to keep prescriptions
- Recall classification system
- Good Manufacturing Practice

Miscellaneous

- Exceptions to child-resistant packaging
- Mailing controlled substances

Make Sure You Know These!

Not all of these are covered in this book because some are state specific – but this is a good list of things to know for the MPJE

- Know time frames for everything
    - When to report to the DEA, DPS, and board
    - How long to keep records
    - How long to keep CE records
- Emergency kits
- Everything on controlled substances
- DEA form numbers
- Know the common definitions, like *adultered* and *misbranded*
- Automated pharmacy systems
- Telepharmacy/remote pharmacy services
- Childproof containers
- Prescribing methadone
- Pharmacy technician ratios and training requirements
- Buying Plan B
- Prescription label requirements
- Changes to a Schedule II prescription
- Counseling requirements
- Drugs that can be prescribed by a therapeutic optometrist
- Pharmacist-intern and pharmacy technician duties
- Reporting professional liability claims
- Preceptor requirements
- Pharmacist administration of vaccines
- Physician dispensing
- Sterile compounding – the different risk levels and expiration dates

The "Golden Rule" for Pharmacy Law

You are required to follow the strictest standard when comparing federal and state law. For example federal law allows 3 different filing systems for prescriptions but Texas only allows 1. Therefore the correct standard to follow is the Texas law.

Also keep all records for a minimum of 2 years.

Acronyms

ACPE – Accreditation Council for Pharmacy Education
ACLS – Advanced Cardiac Life Support
BCLS – Basic Cardiac Life Support
CE – Continuing education
DEA – Drug Enforcement Administration
DPS – Department of Public Safety
FDA – Food and Drug Administration
FPGEC – Foreign Pharmacy Graduate Equivalency Commission
FPGEE – Foreign Pharmacy Graduate Equivalency Examination
GED – General education development
HEPA – High efficiency particulate air
HIPAA – Health Insurance Portability and Accountability Act
IPA – Isopropyl alcohol
ISO – International Organization of Standardization
MPJE – Multistate Pharmacy Jurisprudence Examination
MSA – Metropolitan statistical area
NABP – National Association of Boards of Pharmacy
NAPLEX – North American Pharmacy Licensing Examination
NDC – National drug code
OTC – Over the counter
PALS – Pediatric Advanced Life Support
PIC – Pharmacist-in-charge
PMR – Patient medication record
PTCB – Pharmacy Technician Certification Board
SOP – Standard operating procedure
SWFI – Sterile water for injection
TPN – Total parentral nutrition
USP/NF – United States Pharmacopeia/National Formulary

Section Two: Federal Laws and Rules

Federal Food, Drug, and Cosmetic Act

Purpose: protect the public health by requiring safe, effective, and properly labeled drugs and devices

History

- **1906 Pure Food and Drug Act**
  - Purity standards only; no efficacy requirements
- **1938 Federal Food, Drug, and Cosmetic Act**
  - Safety standards only; no efficacy requirements
- **1951 Durham-Humphrey Amendments**
  - Created OTC and prescription drug categories
- **1962 Kefauver-Harris Amendment**
  - Efficacy requirements
- **1976 Medical Device Amendment**
  - Added regulatory authority over devices
- **1983 Orphan Drug Act**
  - Incentives to create drugs for rare diseases (longer patent life)
- **1984 Drug Price Competition and Patent Restoration Act**
  - Patent holders received 5 years of patent life because of the FDA's process to review drug applications
- **1988 Prescription Drug Marketing Act of 1987**
  - State licensing of wholesale distributors
  - Banned reimportation of prescription drugs
  - Banned sale, trade, or purchase of drug samples
- **1997 FDA Modernization Act**
  - Requires "Rx only" on the prescription legend
- **1999 Over-the-Counter Labeling Requirements**
  - Standardized OTC labeling

Adultered

Refers to the actual makeup or composition of the drug
- Containing any filthy substance
- May have been contaminated in preparation/storage/packaging
- Good manufacturing practices not followed
- Container may contaminate the drug
- Unsafe color additive
- Strength differs from what listed on the label (A 5% difference is okay)
- Misfilled: drug has been substituted

Misbranded

Refers to the drug labeling
- Labeling is false or misleading
- Manufacturer's labeling requirements:
  - Name and address of manufacturer
  - Quantity
  - Generic and brand name of the drug (if applicable)
  - Strength of the drug
  - Information for use
  - Warnings against use
  - Expiration date
- Pharmacist filling a prescription without authorization from prescriber
- Counterfeit drug
- Packaging violates Poison Prevention Packaging Act
- Packaging not containing all the words or statements as required by law

OTC Label Requirements

- Must contain adequate *directions* for use—in comparison, prescription drug labeling must contain adequate *information* for use
- Display panel with name of product
- Name and address of manufacturer/packer/distributor
- Quantity in container
- Cautions and warnings
- Adequate directions for safe and effective use (must be written for a layperson)
- "Drug Facts" must contain
    - Active ingredients
    - Purpose
    - Uses – indications
    - Warnings
    - Directions
    - Other information
    - Inactive ingredients
    - Questions? (optional) followed by telephone number

Other OTC Rules

- Prescribed an OTC but dose is higher than OTC limits: must be written and filled as a prescription
- If an OTC is written as a prescription, then it needs to be filled as a prescription, but a pharmacist can sell an OTC if he or she feels it to be in the best interest of the patient

Recalls

- FDA has no authority to recall drugs, only devices
- **Class I recall** – reasonable probability exposure will cause serious adverse health effects or death

- **Class II recall** – may cause temporary or medically reversible adverse health effects
- **Class III recall** – not likely to cause adverse health effects

Advertising

- Prescription drug advertising – regulated by FDA
- OTC advertising – regulated by Federal Trade Commission
- Pharmacists may advertise
  - Provide pricing information—must include brand/generic name, strength, dosage form, and price charged for a specific quantity
  - Availability of professional services
  - Price stated must include all charges to consumer; mailing and delivery fees may be stated separately

Pregnancy Categories

Category A
Adequate and well-controlled studies have failed to demonstrate a risk to the fetus in the first trimester of pregnancy (and there is no evidence of risk in later trimesters).

Category B
Animal reproduction studies have failed to demonstrate a risk to the fetus, and there are no adequate and well-controlled studies in pregnant women.

Category C
Animal reproduction studies have shown an adverse effect on the fetus, and there are no adequate and well-controlled

studies in humans, but potential benefits may warrant use of the drug in pregnant women despite potential risks.

Category D
There is positive evidence of human fetal risk based on adverse reaction data from investigational or marketing experience or studies in humans, but potential benefits may warrant use of the drug in pregnant women despite potential risks.

Category X
Studies in animals or humans have demonstrated fetal abnormalities and/or there is positive evidence of human fetal risk based on adverse reaction data from investigational or marketing experience, and the risks involved in use of the drug in pregnant women clearly outweigh potential benefits.

Plan B Rules

- Plan B, Plan B One-Step, and their generic versions are allowed to be sold over-the-counter to consumers 17 years and older and available by prescription only for women 16 years and younger
- Only sold in pharmacies/stores staffed by a licensed pharmacist
- Will be kept behind the pharmacy counter because the packaging has both over-the-counter and prescription labeling
- Proof of age via personal identification will be required at time of purchase
- Men may purchase Plan B—the wording is "to consumers 17 years and older"

Section Three: Federal Controlled Substance Laws

Schedule I Controlled Substances

- High potential for abuse
- No currently accepted medical use
- Lack of accepted safety for use under medical supervision
- Examples:
  - Heroin
  - Lysergic acid diethylamide (LSD)
  - Marijuana (cannabis)
  - Peyote
  - 3,4-methylenedioxymethamphetamine ("ecstasy")
- ** Use of peyote by the Native American Church is allowed, but manufacturers and distributors of peyote must be registered

Schedule II Controlled Substances

- High potential for abuse which may lead to severe psychological or physical dependence
- Examples:
  - Narcotics
    - Hydromorphone (Dilaudid®)
    - Methadone (Dolophine®)
    - Meperidine (Demerol®)
    - Oxycodone (OxyContin®)
    - Fentanyl (Sublimaze® or Duragesic®)
  - Stimulants

- Amphetamine (Dexedrine®, Adderall®)
- Methamphetamine (Desoxyn®)
- Methylphenidate (Ritalin®)
  - Others
    - Cocaine
    - Amobarbital
    - Glutethimide
    - Pentobarbital

Schedule III Controlled Substances

- Potential for abuse less than substances in schedules I or II and abuse may lead to moderate or low physical dependence or high psychological dependence
- Examples:
  - Narcotics
    - Combination products containing less than 15 milligrams of hydrocodone per dosage unit (Vicodin®)
    - Products containing not more than 90 milligrams of codeine per dosage unit (Tylenol with codeine®)
  - Products to treat opioid addiction
    - Buprenorphine (Suboxone® and Subutex®)
  - Others
    - Benzphetamine (Didrex®)
    - Phendimetrazine
    - Ketamine
    - Anabolic steroids

Schedule IV Controlled Substances

- Low potential for abuse relative to substances in Schedule III

- Effective 1/11/12: carisoprodol will be Schedule IV
- Examples:
    o Alprazolam (Xanax®)
    o Clonazepam (Klonopin®)
    o Clorazepate (Tranxene®)
    o Diazepam (Valium®)
    o Lorazepam (Ativan®)
    o Midazolam (Versed®)
    o Temazepam (Restoril®)
    o Triazolam (Halcion®)

Schedule V Controlled Substances

- Low potential for abuse relative to substances listed in schedule IV
- Contain limited quantities of certain narcotics
- Generally used for antitussive, antidiarrheal, and analgesic purposes
- Examples
    o Cough preparations containing not more than 200 milligrams of codeine per 100 milliliters or per 100 grams (Robitussin AC® and Phenergan with Codeine®)

DEA Facts

- The U.S. Drug Enforcement Administration (DEA) is a component of the U.S. Department of Justice
- "responsible for enforcing the controlled substances laws and regulations of the United States"

DEA Registration

- All DEA registrants: register every 3 years with DEA form 224 (for pharmacies)
- DEA sends out renewal form 60 days prior to expiration date
- Must notify DEA in writing if have not received renewal form 45 days prior to expiration date

Prescriptions

- Must be for legitimate medical purposes
- Practitioner must be acting in the usual course of their professional practice
- Pharmacists also have a corresponding responsibility with the practitioner for the proper prescribing and dispensing
- Writing a prescription "for office use" is not allowed; practitioner must order directly from a supplier or distributor
- Narcotic prescriptions may not be written for "detoxification treatment" or "maintenance treatment"
- Physicians should not write prescriptions for themselves or family members (but no law against it)
- Practitioners do not need to register with the DEA if they work at a hospital/institution (can use the hospital's DEA number and then the code assigned to them)
- Schedule III–V are allowed 5 refills in the 6 months from the date written

Prescription Requirements

- A prescription must be written in ink or indelible pencil or typewritten and must be manually signed by the practitioner
- A prescription for a controlled substance must include the following information:
  - Date of issue
  - Patient's name and address
  - Practitioner's name, address, and DEA registration number
  - Drug name
  - Drug strength
  - Dosage form
  - Quantity prescribed
  - Directions for use
  - Number of refills (if any) authorized; and
  - Manual signature of prescriber

DEA Registration Numbers

There is an easy formula to determine if a DEA number is valid

- Add the 1st, 3rd, and 5th digits of the DEA number
- Add the 2nd, 4th and 6th digits and multiply by 2
- Add the results of those two calculations
- The last digit from the sum of the first two steps should be the same as the 7th digit in the DEA number
- Example: BF1234563
  - $1 + 3 + 5 = 9$
  - $2 + 4 + 6 = 12 \times 2 = 24$
  - $9 + 24 = 33$
  - So the 7th digit should be "3"
  - Therefore this DEA number is valid

Partial Refills of Schedule III, IV, and V

Partial refills are allowed, provided that each partial filling is dispensed and recorded in the same manner as a refilling (e.g., date refilled, amount dispensed, initials of dispensing pharmacist), the total quantity dispensed in all partial fillings does not exceed the total quantity prescribed, and no dispensing occurs after 6 months past the date of issue.

Refill Authorizations for Schedule III, IV, and V

- Prescriber allowed to orally authorize additional refills
- Not allowed to exceed 5 refills in a 6-month time period from the date the prescription was originally written
- Quantity of each additional refill must be the same as or less than the initial quantity authorized
- New and separate prescription required for any additional quantities above and beyond the "5 refills in 6 months" limit

Data Processing and Storage Requirements

- Pharmacists are allowed to store refill information in a computer
- System must produce a daily hard copy readout of all processed controlled substance refills
- Each individual pharmacist must verify the information is correct and date and sign the hard copy readout
- A logbook may be used instead of the daily hard copy readout, where each pharmacist must sign a statement every day that says the information entered into the computer that day was correct

DEA Form 222

- Required for the sale or transfer of Schedule I or II controlled substances
- Pharmacies may transfer controlled substances to other pharmacies as long as the total amount is up to 5% of the total amount of controlled substances dispensed in a year without having to register as a wholesaler
- Carbon triplicate: Copy 1, Copy 2, and Copy 3
- Each form is numbered serially
- Preprinted with name, address, and registration number of the registrant; the authorized activity; and the schedules of the registrant
  - Cannot be changed
  - In case of changed information, must have new forms made

Completing a DEA Form 222

- Must be completed in ink, indelible pencil, or typewritten
- Only one item per numbered line on the form
  - "One item" means one drug, strength, and package size
- The number of lines completed must be filled in at the bottom of the form
- Name and address of the supplier must be filled in

Who May Sign a DEA Form 222?

- Individual who signed the DEA registration
- Individual who is authorized through the execution of a power of attorney by an individual who signed the DEA registration

Ordering Drugs Using DEA Form 222

- Purchaser fills out the form and submits Copy 1 and 2 to the supplier and keeps Copy 3 for their records
- Supplier fills the order and records on Copy 1 and 2 the number of commercial or bulk containers supplied on each item and the date shipped to purchaser
- Order may be filled in part, with the balance shipped within 60 days of the date on the form
- After 60 days, the order form is no longer valid
- May only be shipped to the address on the form
- Supplier keeps Copy 1 and forwards Copy 2 to the DEA
- When the purchaser receives the shipment, they must note how many containers received on each item and the date received on Copy 3
- Order form may not be filled if it
  - Is not complete, legible, or properly prepared, executed, or endorsed
  - Shows any adulteration, erasure, or change of any description

Emergency Schedule II Prescriptions

- DEA regulations limit an emergency oral prescription to the quantity necessary to treat the patient during the emergency period
- Oral emergency prescriptions must immediately be reduced to writing by the pharmacist and must contain all the information ordinarily required in a prescription, except for the signature of the prescribing individual practitioner
- If the prescribing individual practitioner is not known to the pharmacist, the pharmacist must make a reasonable effort to determine that the oral authorization came from a registered individual

practitioner, which may include a call back to the prescribing individual practitioner and/or other good faith efforts to ensure the practitioner's identity

- An emergency situation is defined as all of the following:
  - o Immediate administration of the controlled substance is necessary for proper treatment
  - o No appropriate alternative treatments are available including non–Schedule II controlled substances
  - o Not reasonably possible for the physician to provide a written prescription prior to dispensing

Transfer of Business

- Notify DEA 14 days prior to transfer
- Day of transfer: complete inventory, which serves as both the closing and opening inventories
- Transferring schedule II – use official DEA 222 order form
- Transferring schedule III–V – separate document with
  - o Name of drug
  - o Dosage form
  - o Strength
  - o Quantity
  - o Date transferred
  - o Names, addresses, and DEA numbers of the pharmacies

Disposing of Controlled Substances by a Reverse Distributor

- May send to a reverse distributor registered with the DEA
  - Schedule II – DEA 222
  - Schedule III–V – written record of name, form, strength, quantity
- Reverse distributor will submit to the DEA form 41 when the controlled substances have been destroyed
- Disposal by those **not** registered with the DEA (ex. long-term care facilities)

Disposing of Controlled Substances at a Pharmacy

- Once a year, retail pharmacies may request DEA permission to dispose of controlled substances that are unwanted, expired, etc.
- Pharmacy completes DEA Form 41 that lists all drugs to be destroyed
- Pharmacy sends letter to DEA with the form at least 14 days in advance, asking for permission
  - Letter contains the proposed date of destruction, method of destruction, and identity of the two witnesses (licensed physician, pharmacist, mid-level practitioner, nurse, or state or local law enforcement officer)

Returning a Controlled Substance Prescription

- An individual may not return unused controlled substance prescription medication to the pharmacy
- There are no provisions in federal laws and regulations to acquire controlled substances from a non-registrant (e.g., individual patient)

- An individual may dispose of their own controlled substance medication without approval from DEA

Theft or Significant Loss
- Notify DEA within one business day of the discovery
- Notify local law enforcement and state regulatory agencies
- Complete DEA form 106

Inventory Requirements
- Actual count of Schedule II
- Estimate count of Schedule III, IV, and V if bottle is <1,000 count
- Actual count of Schedule III, IV, and V if bottle >1,000 count
- Keep records for 2 years
- Records and inventories of Schedule I and II must be kept separately from all other records
- Records and inventories of Schedule III, IV, and V must be kept separately from all other records or readily retrievable
- Inventory of all controlled substances must be done every 2 years

Authorized Agent of the Prescriber
- An authorized agent of the prescriber may
  - Prepare a controlled substance prescription for the signature of the prescriber
  - Orally communicated a prescriber's Schedule III–V prescription to a pharmacist
  - Transmit by fax a prescriber's written Schedule II prescription to a pharmacist
- An authorized agent **cannot** orally communicate an emergency Schedule II prescription to a pharmacist

- To be an agent of the prescriber, a detailed written document must be created and specifies the authority being granted
- DEA also recommends providing a copy to pharmacies likely to receive prescriptions from the prescriber's agent
- Pharmacists still retain responsibility to make sure the controlled substance prescription conforms to the appropriate laws and regulations and is for a legitimate medical purpose

Electronic Prescribing of Controlled Substances
- Practitioners may write electronic controlled substance prescriptions
- Pharmacies may receive, dispense, and archive these electronic prescriptions
- Pharmacies must use specific software approved by the DEA, which must be certified by a third party audit

Central Filling of Controlled Substances
- Central fill pharmacies are permitted to fill the initial and refills of Schedule II, III, IV, and V prescriptions
- May be transmitted electronically or via fax from the community pharmacy
- Community pharmacy writes "CENTRAL FILL" on the face of the original prescription and includes name, address and DEA number of the central fill pharmacy
- Central fill pharmacies must place a label to the packaging showing the local pharmacy name and address as well as a unique identifier to show it was filled at the central fill pharmacy

Prescribing Methadone for Pain

- Federal law and regulations do not restrict the prescribing, dispensing, or administering of any schedule II, III, IV, or V narcotic medication, including methadone, for the treatment of pain, if such treatment is deemed medically necessary by a registered practitioner acting in the usual course of professional practice.
- Use of methadone for the maintenance or detoxification of opioid-addicted individuals, in which case the practitioner is required to be registered with the DEA as a Narcotic Treatment Program (NTP)

Detoxification or Maintenance Treatment

- A practitioner may administer or dispense directly (but not prescribe) a narcotic drug listed in any schedule to a narcotic-dependent person for the purpose of maintenance or detoxification treatment if the practitioner meets both of the following conditions:
    - is separately registered with DEA as a narcotic treatment program
    - complies with DEA regulations regarding treatment qualifications, security, records, and unsupervised use of the drugs
- A physician who is not specifically registered to conduct a narcotic treatment program may administer (but not prescribe) narcotic drugs to a person for the purpose of relieving acute withdrawal symptoms when necessary while arrangements are being made for referral for treatment.
    - No more than 1 day's medication may be administered to the person or for the person's use at one time.

- o Such emergency treatment may be carried out for no more than 3 days and may not be renewed or extended.
- Physicians may administer or dispense narcotic drugs in a hospital to maintain or detoxify a person as an incidental adjunct to a medical or surgical treatment of conditions other than addiction or those with intractable pain

Transferring Controlled Substance Prescriptions

- Allowed one time only
    - o If pharmacies electronically share a real-time, online database, pharmacies may transfer up to the maximum refills permitted
- Must be communicated directly between two licensed pharmacists
- Transferring pharmacist
    - o Voids the prescription
    - o Records the name, address, and DEA number of the pharmacy to which it was transferred
    - o Records the name of the pharmacist receiving the prescription
    - o Records the date of the transfer and name of the pharmacist performing the transfer
- Receiving pharmacist writes
    - o "Transfer" on the face of the prescription
    - o Date of issuance of original prescription
    - o Original number of refills authorized
    - o Date of original dispensing
    - o Number of valid refills remaining and date(s) and locations of previous refill(s)
    - o Pharmacy's name, address, DEA number, and prescription number from which the prescription was transferred

- o Name of pharmacist who transferred the prescription
- o Pharmacy's name, address, DEA number, and prescription number from which the prescription was originally filled

Dispensing Without a Prescription

A controlled substance listed in Schedules II, III, IV, or V which is not a prescription drug as determined under the Federal Food, Drug, and Cosmetic Act, may be dispensed by a pharmacist without a prescription to a purchaser at retail, provided that:

- Only done by a pharmacist and not by a nonpharmacist employee even if under the supervision of a pharmacist (although after the pharmacist has fulfilled his professional and legal responsibilities set forth in this section, the actual cash, credit transaction, or delivery, may be completed by a nonpharmacist)

- Not more than 240 cc. (8 ounces) of any such controlled substance containing opium, nor more than 120 cc. (4 ounces) of any other such controlled substance nor more than 48 dosage units of any such controlled substance containing opium, nor more than 24 dosage units of any other such controlled substance may be dispensed at retail to the same purchaser in any given 48-hour period

- Purchaser is at least 18 years of age

- Pharmacist requires every purchaser of a controlled substance under this section not known to him to furnish suitable identification (including proof of age where appropriate)

- A bound record book for dispensing of controlled substances under this section is maintained by the pharmacist, which book shall contain the name and address of the purchaser, the name and quantity of controlled substance purchased, the date of each purchase, and the name or initials of the pharmacist who dispensed the substance

- A prescription is not required for distribution or dispensing of the substance pursuant to any other Federal, State or local law

- Central fill pharmacies may not dispense controlled substances to a purchaser at retail pursuant to this section.

Section Four: Compounding Sterile Preparations

Personnel

- A pharmacist shall inspect and approve all components, drug preparation containers, closures, labeling, and any other materials involved in the compounding process
- A pharmacist shall review all compounding records for accuracy and conduct checks during and after the compounding process to ensure that errors have not occurred
- A pharmacist shall be accessible at all times to respond to patients' and other health professionals' questions and needs. Such access may be through a telephone or pager which is answered 24 hours a day
- All pharmacy personnel preparing sterile preparations shall receive didactic and experiential training and competency evaluation through
  - Demonstration
  - Testing (written and practical), as outlined by the pharmacist-in-charge and described in the policy and procedure or training manual
- The aseptic technique of each person compounding or responsible for the direct supervision of personnel compounding sterile preparations shall be observed and evaluated as satisfactory through written and practical tests, and media-fill challenge testing, and such evaluation documented
- Although media-fill tests may be incorporated into the experiential portion of a training program, media-fill tests must be conducted at each pharmacy where an

individual compounds sterile preparations. No preparation intended for patient use shall be compounded by an individual until the on-site media-fill tests test indicates that the individual can competently perform aseptic procedures, except that a pharmacist may temporarily compound sterile preparations and supervise pharmacy technicians compounding sterile preparations without media-fill tests provided the pharmacist:

- o Has completed a recognized course in an accredited college of pharmacy or a course sponsored by an ACPE accredited provider that provides 20 hours of instruction and experience in the areas listed in this subparagraph; **and**
- o Completes the on-site media-fill tests within seven (7) days of commencing work at the pharmacy

- Media-fill test procedures for assessing the preparation of specific types of sterile preparations shall be representative of all types of manipulations, products, risk levels, and batch sizes that personnel preparing that type of sterile preparation are likely to encounter
- The pharmacist-in-charge shall ensure continuing competency of pharmacy personnel through in-service education, training, and media-fill tests to supplement initial training. Personnel competency shall be evaluated
  - o During orientation and training prior to the regular performance of those tasks
  - o Whenever the quality assurance program yields an unacceptable result
  - o Whenever unacceptable techniques are observed; **and**

- o   At least on an annual basis for low- and medium-risk level compounding, and every six (6) months for high-risk level compounding

Pharmacists

All pharmacists who compound sterile preparations for administration to patients or supervise pharmacy technicians and pharmacy technician trainees compounding sterile preparations shall complete through a single course, a minimum of 20 hours of instruction and experience. Such training may be obtained through:

- Completion of a structured on-the-job didactic and experiential training program at the pharmacy that provides 20 hours of instruction and experience. Such training may not be transferred to another pharmacy unless the pharmacies are under common ownership and control and use a common training program; **or**
- Completion of a recognized course in an accredited college of pharmacy or a course sponsored by an ACPE accredited provider that provides 20 hours of instruction and experience

Pharmacy Technicians and Pharmacy Technician Trainees

In addition to specific qualifications for registration, all pharmacy technicians and pharmacy technician trainees who compound sterile preparations for administration to patients shall have initial training obtained through completion of a single course, a minimum of 40 hours of instruction

Documentation of Training

The pharmacy shall maintain a record on each person who compounds sterile preparations. The record shall contain, at a minimum, a written record of initial and in-service training, education, and the results of written and practical testing and media-fill testing of pharmacy personnel.

Operational Standards

Sterile preparations may be compounded in licensed pharmacies

- Upon presentation of a practitioner's prescription drug or medication order based on a valid pharmacist/patient/prescriber relationship
- In anticipation of future prescription drug or medication orders based on routine, regularly observed prescribing patterns (see more on this under non-sterile compounding)
- In reasonable quantities for office use by a practitioner and for use by a veterinarian

Any preparation compounded in anticipation of future prescription drug or medication orders shall be labeled

- Name and strength of the compounded preparation **or** list of the active ingredients and strengths
- Facility's lot number
- Beyond-use date
- Quantity or amount in the container
- Appropriate ancillary instructions, such as storage instructions or cautionary statements, including hazardous drug warning labels where appropriate

Other Rules

- Commercially available products – same conditions as non-sterile compounding
- A pharmacy may enter into an agreement to compound and dispense prescription/medication orders for another pharmacy, provided the pharmacy complies with the title relating to Centralized Prescription Dispensing
- Compounding pharmacies/pharmacists may advertise and promote the fact that they provide sterile prescription compounding services, which may include specific drug preparations and classes of drugs
- A pharmacy may not compound veterinary preparations for use in food-producing animals except in accordance with federal guidelines

Microbial Contamination Risk Levels

Risk Levels for sterile compounded preparations shall be as outlined in Chapter 797, Pharmacy Compounding—Sterile Preparations of the USP/NF and as listed below

Low-risk level compounded sterile preparations

- The compounded sterile preparations are compounded with aseptic manipulations entirely within ISO Class 5 or better air quality using only sterile ingredients, products, components, and devices
- The compounding involves only transfer, measuring, and mixing manipulations with closed or sealed packaging systems that are preformed promptly and attentively
- Manipulations are limited to aseptically opening ampules, penetrating sterile stoppers on vials with

sterile needles and syringes, and transferring sterile liquids in sterile syringes to sterile administration devices and packages of other sterile products
- For a low-risk preparation, the storage periods may not exceed the following periods before administration:
  - 48 hours at controlled room temperature
  - 14 days if stored at a cold temperature
  - 45 days if stored in a frozen state, at minus 20 degrees Celsius or colder
  - For delayed activation device systems, the storage period begins when the device is activated

Examples of Low-Risk Compounding
- Single volume transfers of sterile dosage forms from ampules, bottles, bags, and vials; using sterile syringes with sterile needles, other administration devices, and other sterile containers
- Manually measuring and mixing no more than *three (3)* manufactured products to compound drug admixtures

Low-Risk Level compounded sterile preparations with 12-hour or fewer beyond-use date
- The compounded sterile preparations are compounded in compounding aseptic isolator or compounding aseptic containment isolator that is not ISO Class 5 or better or the compounded sterile preparations are compounded in laminar airflow workbench or a biological safety cabinet that cannot be located within an ISO Class 7 buffer area
- Administration of such compounded sterile preparations must commence within 12 hours of preparation or as recommended in the manufacturers' package insert, whichever is less

Medium-risk level compounded sterile preparations

Medium-risk level compounded sterile preparations are those compounded aseptically under low-risk conditions, and one or more of the following conditions exist

- Multiple individual or small doses of sterile products are combined or pooled to prepare a compounded sterile preparation that will be administered either to multiple patients or to one patient on multiple occasions
- The compounding process includes complex aseptic manipulations other than the single-volume transfer
- The compounding process requires unusually long duration, such as that required to complete the dissolution or homogenous mixing (e.g., reconstitution of intravenous immunoglobulin or other intravenous protein products)
- The compounded sterile preparations do not contain broad-spectrum bacteriostatic substances and they are administered over several days (e.g., an externally worn infusion device)
- For a medium-risk preparation, the beyond-use dates may not exceed the following time periods before administration:
  - 30 hours at controlled room temperature
  - 9 days at a cold temperature
  - 45 days in solid frozen state, at minus 20 degrees Celsius or colder

Examples of medium-risk compounding

- Compounding of total parenteral nutrition fluids using a manual or automated device, during which there are multiple injections, detachments, and attachments of nutrient-source products to the device or machine to deliver all nutritional components to a final sterile container

- Filling of reservoirs of injection and infusion devices with multiple sterile drug products, and evacuating air from those reservoirs before the filled device is dispensed
- Filling of reservoirs of injection and infusion devices with volumes of sterile drug solutions that will be administered over several days at ambient temperatures between 25 and 40 degrees Celsius (77 and 104 degrees Fahrenheit)
- Transferring volumes from multiple ampules or vials into a single, final sterile container or product

High-risk level compounded sterile preparations

High-risk level compounded sterile preparations are those compounded under any of the following conditions
- Non-sterile ingredients, including manufactured products, are incorporated; or a non-sterile device is employed before terminal sterilization
- Sterile ingredients, components, devices, and mixtures are exposed to air quality inferior to ISO Class 5.
    - This includes storage in environments inferior to ISO Class 5 of opened or partially used packages of manufactured sterile products that lack antimicrobial preservatives
- Non-sterile preparations are exposed no more than 6 hours before being sterilized
- For a high-risk preparation, the beyond-use dates may not exceed the following time periods before administration:
    - 24 hours at controlled room temperature
    - 3 days at a cold temperature
    - 45 days in solid frozen state, at minus 20 degrees or colder

- All high-risk compounded sterile aqueous solutions subjected to terminal sterilization are passed through a filter with a nominal porosity not larger than 1.2 micron preceding or during filling into their final containers to remove particulate matter. Sterilization of high-risk level compounded sterile preparations by filtration shall be performed entirely within an ISO Class 5 or superior air quality environment

Examples of high-risk compounding

- Dissolving non-sterile bulk drug powders to make solutions, which will be terminally sterilized
- Exposing the sterile ingredients and components used to prepare and package compounded sterile preparations to room air quality worse than ISO Class 5
- Measuring and mixing sterile ingredients in non-sterile devices before sterilization is performed
- Assuming, without appropriate evidence or direct determination, that packages of bulk ingredients contain at least 95% by weight of their active chemical moiety and have not been contaminated or adulterated between uses

Immediate Use Compounded Sterile Preparations

For the purpose of emergency or immediate patient care, such situations may include cardiopulmonary resuscitation, emergency room treatment, preparation of diagnostic agents, or critical therapy where the preparation of the compounded sterile preparation under low-risk level conditions would subject the patient to additional risk due to delays in therapy. Compounded sterile preparations are exempted from the requirements described in this paragraph for low-risk, medium-risk, and high-risk level compounded sterile preparations when all of the following criteria are met.

- Only simple aseptic measuring and transfer manipulations are performed with not more than three (3) sterile non-hazardous commercial drug and diagnostic radiopharmaceutical drug products, including an infusion or diluent solution
- Unless required for the preparation, the preparation procedure occurs continuously without delays or interruptions and does not exceed 1 hour
- Administration begins not later than one (1) hour following the completion of preparing the compounded sterile preparation
- When the compounded sterile preparations is not administered by the person who prepared it or its administration is not witnessed by the person who prepared it, the compounded sterile preparation shall bear a label listing patient identification information such as name and identification number(s), the names and amounts of all ingredients, the name or initials of the person who prepared the compounded sterile preparation, and the exact 1-hour beyond-use time and date
- If administration has not begun within one (1) hour following the completion of preparing the compounded sterile preparation, the compounded sterile preparation is promptly and safely discarded. Immediate-use compounded sterile preparations shall not be stored for later use
- Cytotoxic drugs shall not be prepared as immediate-use compounded sterile preparations

Environment

A pharmacy that prepares low- and medium-risk preparations shall have a clean room/controlled area for the compounding of sterile preparations that is constructed to minimize the opportunities for particulate and microbial contamination. The clean room/controlled area shall

- Contain an anteroom/ante-zone that provides at least an ISO Class 8 air quality
- Contain a buffer zone or buffer room designed to maintain at least ISO Class 7 conditions

The pharmacy shall prepare sterile pharmaceuticals in a primary engineering control device, such as a laminar air flow hood, biological safety cabinet, compounding aseptic isolator, compounding aseptic containment isolator which is capable of maintaining at least ISO Class 5 conditions during normal activity. The isolator must provide isolation from the room and maintain ISO Class 5 during dynamic operating conditions, including transferring ingredients, components, and devices into and out of the isolator and during preparation of compounded sterile preparations

Cytotoxic Drugs

- All personnel involved in the compounding of cytotoxic products shall wear appropriate protective apparel, such as gowns, face masks, eye protection, hair covers, shoe covers or dedicated shoes, and appropriate gloving
- Cytotoxic drugs shall be prepared in a Class II or III vertical flow biological safety cabinet or compounding aseptic containment isolator located in an ISO Class 7 area that is physically separated from other preparation areas
- Compounding area must have negative air pressure compared to the anteroom, which must have positive air pressure

Cleaning and Disinfecting the Sterile Compounding Areas

- Shall be conducted prior to and after each work shift (at a minimum of every 12 hours while the pharmacy is open) and when there are spills
- Before compounding is performed, all items are removed from the direct and contiguous compounding areas and all surfaces are cleaned of loose material and residue from spills, followed by an application of a residue-free disinfecting agent (e.g., IPA), that is left on for a time sufficient to exert its antimicrobial effect
- Work surfaces near the direct and contiguous compounding areas in the buffer or clean area are cleaned of loose material and residue from spills, followed by an application of a residue-free disinfecting agent that is left on for a time sufficient to exert its antimicrobial effect
- Floors in the buffer or clean area are cleaned by mopping at least once daily when no aseptic operations are in progress
- In the anteroom area, walls, ceilings, and shelving shall be cleaned monthly
- Supplies and equipment removed from shipping cartons must be wiped with a disinfecting agent, such as IPA. No shipping or other external cartons may be taken into the buffer or clean area
- Storage shelving, emptied of all supplies, walls, and ceilings are cleaned and disinfected at least monthly

Personnel Cleansing and Garbing

- Any person with an apparent illness or open lesion that may adversely affect the safety or quality of a drug preparation being compounded shall be excluded from direct contact with components, drug preparation containers, closures, any materials involved in the compounding process, and drug products until the condition is corrected

- Before entering the clean area, compounding personnel must remove the following:
  - o personal outer garments (e.g., bandanas, coats, hats, jackets, scarves, sweaters, vests)
  - o all cosmetics, because they shed flakes and particles; **and**
  - o all hand, wrist, and other body jewelry
- Artificial nails or extenders are prohibited while working in the sterile compounding environment
- Personnel must don personal protective equipment and perform hand hygiene in an order that proceeds from the dirtiest to the cleanest activities as follows:
  - o Shoe covers
  - o Head and facial hair covers
  - o Face mask
  - o Wash hands and arms up to elbows – minimum 30 seconds
  - o Gown
  - o Gloves
  - o 70% IPA to gloves (and routinely during compounding)
- When taking a break – the gown may be stored in the anteroom and reused, but shoe covers, hair and facial hair covers, face mask, and gloves must be replaced, and hand hygiene must be performed

Section Five: Pseudoephederine Laws

- Sold for personal use through face-to-face stores, mobile retail vendors, or through the mail
- Nonliquid (includes gelcaps) forms **must** be in unit dose packaging
- Report losses to the DEA (examples: theft, in-transit)
- Max of 3.6 grams per day per purchaser
- Max of 7.5 grams per 30-day period per purchaser at a mobile retail vendor
- Customers may not have direct access to the products (e.g., store behind counter or in locked case)
- Seller must maintain a written (bound record book) or electronic list of each sale, including
    - Name of product
    - Quantity sold
    - Name of purchaser
    - Address of purchaser
    - Date and time of sale
    - Signature of purchaser
- Seller must keep the logbook for at least 2 years from the date of sale
- Each seller must do a self-certification with the DEA
- Sales personnel must be trained

Resources/Bibliography

NAPLEX®/MPJE® – www.nabp.net

MPJE® Registration Bulletin
http://www.nabp.net/programs/assets/NAPLEX-MPJE.pdf

Electronic Prescriptions for Controlled Substances
http://www.deadiversion.usdoj.gov/ecomm/e_rx/faq/pharmacies.htm

Federal Food, Drug, and Cosmetic Act
http://www.access.gpo.gov/uscode/title21/chapter9_.html

Federal Controlled Substance Act
http://www.deadiversion.usdoj.gov/21cfr/cfr/index.html

Poison Prevention Packaging Act
http://www.cpsc.gov/cpscpub/pubs/384.pdf

10479278R00037

Made in the USA
San Bernardino, CA
15 April 2014